Non - Diabetic Hypoglycaemia - On the Way to a Cure

by

Rachel Henderson

Non-Diabetic Hypoglycaemia – On the Way to a Cure

by

Rachel Henderson

Non-Diabetic Hypoglycaemia – On the Way to a Cure

Copyright Notice

First Published in 2011 in Great Britain by Bowbridge Publishing, 18 Bowbridge Lock, Stroud, Gloucestershire, GL5 2JZ, UK

http://www.bowbridgepublishing.com

info@bowbridgepublishing.com

Contents

About the Author

Hi, I am Rachel. I was diagnosed with hypoglycaemia when I was a few months old as my mother mentioned to her doctor that I got 'shaky' when I was hungry. He told her that I would benefit from having glucose drinks if this happened.

I then grew up being a very shy and nervous person on the normal childhood diet of that time, potatoes, crisps, sweets, chocolate, cakes, biscuits and puddings. I was given glucose when I showed signs of low blood sugar. When I reached adulthood, there was a lot more information about hypoglycaemia around and I bought some books from America, which changed the way I saw my condition and treated it.

After learning more about the condition and how to treat it, I then changed my diet drastically. I cut out sugar completely and moved to wholemeal. It was a big change but I was aware of how much difference it could make and so I was prepared to try it. I found that I become less nervous and shy and I also felt a lot better in myself. As I learnt more about the glycaemic index I altered what I was eating and then again after doing a nutrition course with The Open University. I felt like I was refining my diet more and more so that not only was it healthy and balanced but it was also keeping by blood sugar levels as stable as possible.

I am not a perfect eater and still get hormonal moments when I feel the need to consume my body weight in chocolate and I cannot always resist cravings. Sometimes I have to have white rice or I have a slice of cake, but I aware of what it does to me and why it is a good idea, not to have it too often. M understanding of my condition and how food relates to it makes my quality of life much better.

I now understand my symptoms better and when my body is asking for food. I know what to eat when I get those symptoms too. I also know my body and work hard to ignore the cravings for sugar and eat foods that are better for me.

I am now a more confident person and do not get nervous so often and am certainly no longer shy. I am less temperamental and I have a lot more energy.

Introduction

Hypoglycaemia is a disease which many people suffer from. It is something which many doctors do not recognise, or only as a precursor of diabetes or a symptom of too much insulin in diabetes. However, it is a condition in its own right, causing a variety of different symptoms in different people, which is why it can be very difficult to diagnose.

However, treatment is solely by diet and lifestyle changes and so they can be achieved without a diagnosis and the great thing is that the recommended diet is a healthy, balanced diet and so something that is recommended by doctors and dieticians anyway.

Many people experience feeling moody if they are late with a meal or they get headaches when they eat a lot of sugar. These are the symptoms of low blood sugar. Some people find that they get very badly affected when they get an episode of low blood sugar and some do not.

If you suffer from tiredness, irritability when you skip a meal or are generally not feeling well, then it could be possible that you have low blood sugar. It might, therefore, be worth having an attempt at changing your diet in order to see whether you feel better.

What Does Hypoglycaemia Mean?

Hypoglycaemia is a condition in the body when the amount of sugar in the blood stream is lower than the level the body needs. This means that it does not have the energy required to function properly. It can therefore make you feel tired, but there are many other symptoms too. If you never eat regularly and you suffer from low blood sugar then you may find that you have the symptoms all of the time and so you may not notice that there is anything in particular wrong with you. You may just think that you are prone to feeling unwell. Sometimes the symptoms can disappear as well, especially if you do get low blood sugar often. This can be dangerous because if it gets too low it can be serious and if you do not notice the symptoms, there is a chance that it will get low and it will be too late when you notice.

It is possible with short term hypoglycaemia, for anyone to get it. If you do not eat for a long time, then your body will be deficient in sugars and you will see the symptoms. However, some people seem to be much more prone to it than others. There are a variety of reasons why this might be; it sometimes seems to run in families, for example. It also can be caused by problems with the pancreas. It can be wise to see a doctor to rule out any serious causes, but they are only likely to take you seriously if you have symptoms which have started recently, rather than always having them.

Symptoms

There are many different symptoms of hypoglycaemia and some people get a lot of them and others get just a few.

If you normally eat regularly and you skip a meal, then you may experience some of the symptoms. You could find that you are shaky, irritable and tired. You may feel sick and not feel like eating and you may get a headache and even feel thirsty.

If you tend not to eat regularly or eat well, then you may have more long term symptoms. These are things like always tired, insomnia, nervous disposition, irritable or having mood swings, temperamental, low energy, headaches, aching muscles,

It is always wise to visit the doctor before you undertake any lifestyle change. It can be very tempting to self-diagnose with the Internet giving us so much health information. However, because the symptoms are so common, they could be due to other things or the low blood sugar could be a side effect of another disorder and so it is wise to get it checked out. It is good to eliminate any other illnesses or diseases first. Tell them your symptoms and they may decide to run some tests and things like that. The doctor may not diagnose hypoglycaemia though and this is because many do not recognise it as a disorder in its own right. However, if you have eliminated other possibilities, then you can at least relax knowing that it is not anything nasty. Then you can have a go at altering your diet as it will not hurt you. You could check with them first.

If you already have any medical conditions and are on medication, then you will need to speak to your doctor about your proposed change of diet. If you are changing your exercise routine, it could be important to mention that to them as well.

It is possible that the symptoms stop showing after a while, although the blood sugar levels are still low. This happens because the brain gets use to being in a state of low blood sugar. If you have any suspicions that you have low blood sugar, then you may as well have a go at the diet and see how it affects you. It should make you feel more energetic and healthier, you may not realise how unwell you have felt until you change your habits to healthier ones and then you will certainly notice a difference.

A list of symptoms follows. You may find you only get a few or all of them, it does vary from person to person:

Headache

Sensitivity to light

Palpitations

Not wanting to be touched

Outbursts of temper

Stressed

Non-Diabetic Hypoglycaemia – On the Way to a Cure

Tired / nodding off in day

Cannot sleep

Nightmares

Craving food and hunger

Sickness or nausea and stomach ache

Shaking

Irritable

Shy/nervous

Daydreamy

Blurred vision

Dilated pupils

Flashes of light in the vision

Fainting

Hyperactive

Sweating and hot

Cold and clammy

Incoordination

Coma or seizures

Symptoms also depend on the part of the body that is affected by the lack of sugar in the blood. Some are caused by the hormones that try to work to reverse the effects of the low blood sugar. These are adrenaline and glucagon. The others are from the brain being affected by low amounts of sugar. The Adrenaline produces shakiness, sweating and palpitations. The glucagon reduces hunger, sickness and headache. The lack of sugar in the brain leads to the emotional changes and can also cause tiredness, dizziness, blurred and double vision, slurred speech, seizures and coma. You can get all the symptoms at once, just a few of them or only ones associated with one of the causes. Of course, you may get some of the symptoms, when you have not got low blood sugar. For example you could easily get sweaty, palpitations and shakiness due to stress causing adrenaline and it may not necessarily then lead to low blood sugar, although there is a chance that it might do.

The symptoms can occur in a different order and some may never appear or not every time. Children may have different symptoms to adults. For example, young children might be sick, older ones seem like they are drunk and in the elderly the symptoms may even resemble a stroke. The symptoms may change because of how often the blood sugar is getting low and also how quickly the blood sugar drops. If the blood sugar keeps dropping then it could cause damage to the body as well.

Long term hypoglycaemia can be found to lead to more serious medical conditions. The increase in adrenalin can lead to high blood pressure and even heart attacks. Some people find they get depression. It is therefore important to sort things out before it all gets very serious.

Controlling Blood Sugar

Many people would automatically think that if you suffer from low blood sugar, then the way to control it would be to eat sugar. In fact it was even something that doctors used to recommend. However, this is the worst thing that can be done in most cases. If you have passed out, or are about to, then it could be worth doing this to bring you back round, but you will then need to eat something which will release energy more slowly, to avoid another dip in blood sugar. Something like a slice of wholemeal toast would be ideal.

When you eat pure sugar, the blood sugar levels in the blood increase. The pancreas releases the hormone insulin which reduces the blood sugar level and takes it to a more normal amount. However, if you suffer from hypoglycaemia, it is likely that the pancreas will over react and produces too much insulin. This will cause the blood sugar levels to fall lower than normal and it produces some of the symptoms listed above. The spikes in blood sugar can be difficult for anyone to cope with because the high sugar levels can give you a rush of energy and then as it drops, even to a normal level you miss that feeling and notice the drop in energy. It is therefore best to try to stabilise the blood sugar level so that it remains normal all of the time.

This can be quite difficult; some people find it harder than others, depending on the severity of their condition. The first thing to do is to avoid spikes in blood sugar.

Diet

Therefore you need to work hard at changing your diet. If you make a huge change and cut out all the foods that are bad for your blood sugar and include the good things, you will notice an immediate and huge difference. However, this is not always easy to do and a step by step approach can be easier to get used to. This could involve substituting one bad item each week, so replacing sweets with fruit in the first week and then continuing with this in the second week but also changing to wholemeal bread.

You will know whether you can manage a big change or whether small ones will be better for you. You will also know which changes will be easiest and which will not. Take a look at the foods that you should and should not eat and it will help you to decide what might be easy to do and what might not. Then you can perhaps do several easy things to start with and then gradually do the harder things.

Exercise

Too much exercise can lead to a big drop in blood sugar. Athletes tend to drink sugary drinks to keep them energised, but unless you are training for some big event, it is better to have foods which give you energy for longer. Snack on fruit or even sandwiches and try to avoid the big sugar spike you get from energy and sports drinks. Take things easy and do not do too much either as this could make the blood sugar drop.

It is worth experimenting with exercise to find out what suits you. You may find that exercising for short period's suits you better or that a longer period of lower impact exercise works better. It is worth trying different things; you may even find that exercising at a certain time of the day is more effective. It should not put you off exercise though. Everyone needs to exercise and so it is important to make sure that you find something that you can do.

Stress

Stress can be a big factor in blood sugar. Low blood sugar causes the release of adrenalin which causes stress which causes the body to release adrenalin which causes the blood sugar to lower. This is a vicious circle and things can get very bad. If you manage your diet, then this could really help, but it is also important to try to find a way of managing the stress. Try relaxation techniques, there are many that you can try out for free, you can find out about them online. Try to avoid stress as much as you can as well, if this is possible.

It is good to perhaps consider yoga classes or meditation. Try to find some techniques which you can apply when a stressful situation occurs.

Foods and Hypoglycaemia

Sugar

Avoiding having foods high in sugar can help to reduce the blood sugar spikes. Sugar, in its pure form, as most people know, is found in sweets, chocolate, cakes and biscuits. However, it is also found in jams, chutneys, sauces, ready meals, breakfast cereals and all manner of things. If you start checking food labels, you will be shocked to find how high the sugar levels are in many foods. In fact, it can be difficult to avoid having any sugar at all.

There are many hidden sugars as well, reading the ingredients does not always clearly show them. Pure sugars end in -ose so glucose, sucrose, fructose, lactose, maltose etc. are all forms of sugar. Glucose is the purest form of sugar, sucrose is what we commonly refer to as sugar (granulated, caster, icing sugar are all sucrose), fructose is sugar from fruit. Also syrup, honey and treacle are almost completely sugar.

It can be very difficult to completely avoid sugar, but if you can cut it down a lot, then this can make a big difference. However, there are ways that you can have a bit of sugar and cancel out the effects. This will be explained later in the section on Glycaemic Index.

Many people worry about cutting out sugar completely. They think that it is something that the body needs. It is true, the body does need sugar, but it can make sugar from the foods you eat and so it is never necessary to have it in the pure form.

Carbohydrates

All forms of carbohydrate have some sugar in. They come with different forms of sugar. These are things like flour, pastry, pasta, rice, potatoes, biscuits, bread and cakes. Fruit and vegetables also contain carbohydrates. These items tend to make up part of our staple diet and so are not things we would consider eliminating. In fact we need carbohydrates to give us energy and cutting them out is not a sensible thing to do.

There are forms of carbohydrate which are broken down more easily than others. Those that can be broken down easily produce a blood sugar spike because we get a rush of sugar, followed by nothing. Things that are broken down more slowly, cause a slowly energy release and so not only does the energy last longer, we do not get that big sugar rush. Sometimes how we cook an item can even make a difference to this.

For example, a new potato boiled in its skin until it is just soft is much harder for the body to break down than a jacket potato which has been cooked for several hours. This is because the starches have been broken down in to sugar and the body has to work less hard to do this. Cooking anything for less time or even it raw (in the case of fruit and vegetables) will make it harder for the body to break down and therefore cause a slower release in energy.

Some fruits can be worse for blood sugar than others. Fruit juice is very easy for the body to turn in to sugar and so is not a good choice. Melon is very sugary as are grapes and dried fruits. Although a good variety of fruits should be included in the diet, to keep you healthy, it can be a good idea to have these less often and stick to apples and pears which are harder for the body to break down. Bananas can also be quite good and soft fruits. Some people are more sensitive than others to the sugars and so it can be a good idea to experiment and cut some out and then reintroduce them and see if they make you feel unwell. Cooked fruit is not so good for blood sugar levels because the sugars have been broken down during the cooking process. However, if you have a very sweet tooth and are trying to wean yourself off sugar, having dried and cooked fruit and fruit juice, can be a good replacement initially, although you should plan to eventually cut these down to a minimum as you get used to the changes.

Vegetables do contain some sugars. However, they have less than fruit and they are harder to break down. We know that we should have a good variety of vegetables and you should not find that you are that sensitive to the sugars in them. However, it can be worth experimenting as some sweeter ones like sweet potatoes, tomatoes and peppers may cause reactions, whereas it is less likely from greens and beans.

With the goods that contain flour, having wholemeal or granary will be harder to break down than white and so it is a good idea to swap to wholemeal flour, bread and pasta and brown rice. It can be best to avoid sweets and to choose biscuits and cakes which have whole grains, added nuts and seeds or lower sugar content.

White Foods

Any processed carbohydrates tend to be white, things like pastry, pizza bases, pasta, rice and bread. These tend to be staples in most peoples diet. Perhaps white toast for breakfast with corn flakes, a pizza and garlic bread for lunch and white rice as part of the evening meal. All of these are very high in easily absorbed sugars and so can be very harmful to blood glucose.

Changing these to less refined products can really help. It can be difficult in some cases. Getting used to the flavour of wholemeal bread and brown rice as well as brown pasta can be an issue for some people and the texture is different as well. However, with some experimentation with combining new flavours and things like that, you may find you actually start to prefer these. It can take time and you may decide to go back to the white versions occasionally.

Cooking with wholemeal flour can be quite difficult. There are a lot of recipes which use it though and it is a good idea to use a recipe specifically including it, rather than adapting a recipe that uses white because it may not work so well. Sieving the flour can help and you may need to add extra liquid or rising agents.

Alcohol

Alcohol can have very bad consequences for those with hypoglycaemia. Alcohol can contain a lot of sugar for one thing. However, it also has bad effects in the body. The body naturally should maintain a level blood sugar. However, when it is concentrating on eliminating the toxins from the alcohol is less efficient at stabilizing the blood sugar. Excessive drinking can even permanently reduce the effectiveness of insulin and blood sugar levels can be higher than normal. However, even drinking small amounts can increase insulin production and cause low blood sugar.

Fats and Protein

Fat and protein do not make blood sugar levels spike up. In fact they are harder to break down and so they really help to stabilize blood sugar. It is important, though, not to have too much fat, especially saturated fat. If you are suffering badly from low blood sugar, then it could be good to increase the fat in the diet for a while, however, it is best to try to find low fat protein sources, which also stabilise blood sugar. Things like low fat dairy, chicken, fish, beans, seeds and small portions of nuts can all help.

Caffeine

Caffeine is found in tea and coffee as well as in smaller amounts in chocolate and in large amounts in certain fizzy drinks. It is something which can cause many of the symptoms of low blood sugar such as shaking. The caffeine causes a rise in adrenaline which is why it makes you feel more alert.

Caffeine also raises blood sugar level slightly; it is possible that the hypoglycaemic may then produce insulin to lower that blood glucose. As they are prone to producing too much insulin, they will be likely to cause a reduction in blood sugar.

It is therefore best to drink drinks which are decaffeinated. It is easy to find decaffeinated tea and coffee and many fizzy drinks do not have caffeine. Chocolate only has small amounts of caffeine, but because of the sugar content it is best avoided anyway.

A Healthy Balanced Diet

We have often heard that a healthy balanced diet is the way to live our lives. It can be difficult to know exactly what this means, but if you follow it, with just a few extra modifications, then you should be able to reduce your hypoglycaemic symptoms.

A balanced diet is one where you have a small amount of fat and sugar, lots of fruits and vegetables, some protein and carbohydrate. An average meal should have half a plate of vegetables, a quarter of a plate of protein and a quarter of a plate of carbohydrates. If you can make the carbohydrates wholemeal, keep the protein low fat and have different vegetables, then you are doing well. For breakfast have whole meal toast or a whole grain cereal with not much added sugar, this would be something like porridge, sugar free muesli, shredded wheat or Weetabix. You need 2-3 portions of fruit a day as well, so you could have those in between meals, if you like to snack or with breakfast or as puddings. It can be a good idea to snack between meals though, to keep your blood sugar more balanced.

If you want more information on what a healthy balanced diet, then your doctor should be able to help you and they might even be able to give you some meal plans and recipes.

Food Supplements

Many people worry about getting enough nutrients and take food supplements to ensure they are healthy. The problem with these is that they are not properly monitored in the UK. The items are not clearly labelled and so it can be hard to know exactly what you are buying.

People should be able to get all the nutrients they need from a healthy balanced diet. Some minerals are said to be good for stabilising blood sugar, but if you have a tendency for low blood sugar, then stabilising it at a low level, is not helpful.

Replacing Foods

Sometimes it can be difficult to imagine what foods you may or may not be able to eat. So below is a list of foods that are not good for blood sugar with a healthier alternative:

White bread – Wholemeal Bread

White Pasta – Wholemeal pasta

White Rice – Brown Rice

Sweets – blueberries/strawberries/raspberries

Sponge pudding and custard – stewed fruit crumble made with wholemeal flour or oats and no added sugar

Chocolate biscuits – wholegrain digestives or oatcakes

Cream Crackers – bran based crackers or oatcakes

Rice Cakes – wholegrain rice cakes

Jam – all fruit jam/marmite/peanut butter

Crisps – Nuts

Roast Potatoes / chips – New potatoes in their skin

Pizza – home-made pizza with wholemeal base

Chocolate cake – wholemeal scone

Sugary tea/coffee – unsweetened drinks

Fizzy drinks – milky unsweetened drinks or water

Cornflakes/rice krispies/special K – porridge, Weetabix, shredded wheat

Trifle – fruit with natural yoghurt

Dried fruit – fresh or tinned fruit

It can be tempting to replace sugar with sweetener. This can help you in the short term but it is not recommended for long term use. The reason is that when something sweet goes in to the mouth, the brain expects to get an energy boost. Sugar does provide that and sweetener will not. It can give you a tendency to then crave foods that will give you that energy anyway. There are also some people that feel that sweeteners are not healthy, there is not a great deal of evidence about this at the moment but it could be something that you want to consider.

There are selections of foods which say that they are low sugar versions, such as tomato ketchup and baked beans and they have sweeteners in. There are some which are sweetened with fruit juice instead. Whichever, you look at, you will find that they are expensive and it could be worth considering using the normal one but in lower quantities or cutting it out altogether. It really depends on how sensitive your body is to the sugar and how much you want to eat those foods.

The Glycaemic Index

The glycaemic index is a list of foods, each with a score. For example glucose scores 100 which is the worst possible score. The aim is to have things which are nearer to zero which would be things like meat, beans, dairy, eggs and fats. However if you combine white rice which scores highly with kidney beans which score low, you could get a better average score for the meal. It is still best to try to avoid the sugars as much as you can, but because carbohydrate is a healthy part of our diet and cannot be avoided and then it can be combined instead, so we get the health benefits, without the unhealthy blood sugar spike and subsequent drop.

Meal Plans

Planning meals can be very important. The combination of foods that you eat can have a big effect on your blood sugar. This is not a complex food combining thing like the diets that are around. This is just making sure that you have proteins or fats with the carbohydrates. These will take the bod longer to digest and can offset the drop in sugar levels you get after the spike when eating carbohydrates. It can be a case of trial and error, but looking at the glycaemic index can help a lot.

The following daily meal plans have been put together with this in mind. Quantities are often vague, because it will depend on whether you are male or female, your age, size and level of fitness as to how many calories you should have in a day. Therefore it is up to you to consider what a good portion size might be.

Non-Diabetic Hypoglycaemia – On the Way to a Cure

Day 1

Porridge cooked with semi-skimmed milk with a banana chopped in to it

An apple and small slice of cheese

Wholegrain seeded bread with ham and lettuce in a sandwich with crudities of carrots, cucumber & peppers

A small handful of mixed nuts

Salmon and dill sauce on wholemeal pasta with peas and mange tout

Buttered bran crackers

Day 2

A slice of wholegrain toast with a poached egg

A banana and some almonds

Wholemeal couscous with roasted vegetables and houmous

A pear with wholegrain rice cakes

Roast chicken with new potatoes, cauliflower cheese, carrots and parsnips

Weetabix with semi-skimmed milk

Day 3

Shredded wheat and semi-skimmed milk

A handful of toasted seeds

Left over roast chicken in a cold salad with wholemeal croutons

2 Satsuma's or small oranges with Brazil nuts

Prawn curry with vegetables and brown rice

A mixture of soft fruits (blueberries, strawberries, blackberries, raspberries) and whole grain biscuits

Day 4

Sugar Free Muesli with semi-skimmed milk with grated apple added in

Peaches with plain yoghurt

Cold new potatoes, scotch egg and green salad

Slice of whole grain toast with peanut butter

Beef stew with wholemeal flour dumplings

Oatcakes

Day 5

Beans on toast

Stewed plums with crumble made from wholemeal flour, oats and cinnamon (no sugar)

Bulgur wheat salad with peppers, tomatoes, cucumber, basil and herbs

Carrot sticks and dips

Wholemeal pasta with tomato and cheese sauce served with roasted Mediterranean vegetables

Mango with natural yoghurt

The meals and snacks can be mixed up, but be sure to have 2-3 portions of fruits a day and 3-5 vegetables. These are just guidelines to give you ideas on what sorts of foods to eat and when. You may have noticed that there are three meals and three snacks a day. The idea behind this is that if you eat often, then it keeps the blood sugar more even. So topping up your energy levels regularly can really help you to feel much better. You do need to be careful though, if you are not used to snacking, you could put on weight and so you need to cut down your portion sizes of your main meal to allow for the extra calories you are eating in between.

It is also important to combine foods that take longer to break down with carbohydrates. This is why the meals all have some protein in. Then the blood sugar should stay more level. Therefore combining fruits with nuts or yoghurt, biscuits with cheese or butter and pasta with meat or fish is a great thing to do.

Sometimes eating too much can cause hypoglycaemia. Eating lots of the wrong foods can cause an energy slump before you have even finished eating a meal. It does sometimes seem that certain foods take so much energy to digest that you get tired after eating. This seems to happen most with stodgy carbohydrate laden meals such as a roast dinner with sponge pudding. It may be more likely to happen if you have gone a long time without eating beforehand. Watch out if this happens to you and avoid this type of meal, if you can.

Recipes

Fruity Porridge

150ml milk

25g porridge

30g sultanas

25g dried apricots

This is again a recipe which uses dried fruit. The slow release energy from the milk and oats should stop them causing a bad reaction, but it is worth experimenting. The fruit saves the need to put sugar in the porridge.

Chop the apricots and put all of the ingredients in a microwavable bowl. Cook for 2 minutes of high power, stir and serve.

Muesli

25g porridge oats

25g chopped cashew nuts

50ml milk

2 tbsp natural yoghurt

Blueberries and raspberries

Stir the porridge in to the milk and then mix in the cashew nuts. Put the yoghurt on top and decorate with the blueberries and raspberries

Roasted Vegetable Lasagne (serves 4)

200g wholemeal lasagne

For the roasted vegetables:

1 red pepper

1 onion

3 cloves garlic

1 yellow pepper

1 courgette

Chop all the vegetables and place in an oven dish with a layer of oil on the bottom. Sir and roast in a preheated 200 degree oven for an hour or until they start to brown.

For the tomato sauce:

A small box passata

1 tbsp tomato paste

1 onion

1 clove garlic

Olive oil

To make the tomato sauce, finely chop the onion and garlic in a food processor and then fry slowly in a tablespoon of olive oil until soft. Then add the passata and tomato paste and bring to the boil. Simmer for 30 minutes.

For the cheese sauce:

1 knob butter

1 teaspoon plain wholemeal flour

½ pint milk

100g grated cheese

Salt & pepper

To make the cheese sauce melt the butter in a saucepan and then add the flour. Using a whisk, add the milk slowly until you get a smooth sauce. Simmer for 3 minutes and then add in the cheese and season to taste

Start the lasagne with a layer of tomato sauce and then place some sheets of the lasagne on top. Then put a layer of cheese sauce, some vegetables and then more lasagne sheets. Keep layering up, finishing with a layer of cheese sauce. Bake in a 200 degree oven for 30 minutes, until the top starts to go golden brown.

Roast Chicken Salad (serves 2)

100g chicken in pieces

1 cos lettuce

Cucumber

Mayonnaise

Croutons

This salad is great for using up leftover roast chicken as it just needs roughly chopped pieces. It can be served with hot, freshly cooked chicken or cold meat. To make the croutons, use a crust of wholemeal bread and cut in to squares. Fry in olive oil until golden brown or for a healthier option, put in the oven with no fat. Leave to cool.

Then roughly chop the lettuce, and cut slices of cucumber and then halve them. Place in a bowl and then sprinkle over the chicken then the croutons. Dress with mayonnaise or Caesar dressing.

Rice Salad (serves 2)

100g brown basmati rice

1 onion

1 red pepper

50g peas

100g chick peas

Olive oil

Boil the brown rice according to the packet instructions, adding a stock cube in to the water. Finely chop the onion and fry in a little olive oil until soft. Finely chop the red pepper and add in with the onion and cook for five minutes. Add in the peas and chick peas and cook for another five minutes and then add in the cooked and drained rice. Serve hot or cold.

Vegetable Soup and Bread

1 onion

1 carrot

1 tin chickpeas

50g peas

1 stock cube

Crusty wholegrain granary bread

Chop the onion and carrot. Put in a saucepan with the chickpeas, peas and stock cube and any other left over vegetables you have. Bring to the boil and simmer for ten minutes. Blend until smooth and serve with the bread warmed up and plenty of butter.

Boiled Fruit Cake

100g sultanas

50g dried chopped apricots

50g dates

50g chopped mixed nuts

100ml apple juice

3 eggs

200g wholemeal flour

100g margarine

1 tbsp mixed spice (optional)

This cake does have dried fruit in, which some hypoglycaemics cannot tolerate. However, if you have to have cake, then this can be a good alternative to other, less healthy options. It is a good idea to have this after a meal, rather than as a snack as then it will be more balanced by the other food.

Warm the apple juice in a saucepan with the sultanas, apricots and spice and simmer for 5 minutes. Mix the margarine with a mixer until smooth and then add in the eggs one at a time with a few spoonfuls of the flour. Once all the flour is added, put in the nuts and the fruit mixture. Put in to a cake tin and bake for 60 minutes at 180 degrees until a skewer comes out clean.

Putting it all together

This selection of recipes and meal plans should give you an idea to build on with regards to meals. It can be quite difficult; to plan out each meal making sure it has protein and carbohydrates and includes enough vegetables so that you get your five a day. However, once you have done it for a while, you will get used to it and it will get easier.

It can be good to start off with a selection of eating plans for a day. So you perhaps have ten days worth of meals and then mix them up as you choose. It may seem a bit dull, but it can be better for you to see what works and what does not, if you stick to a set selection of foods for a while.

It is important to remember that food is fuel and energy and nutrients and that is all it should be. It is tempting to think of certain foods as treats or fun to eat but this is the route to being unhealthy. Unfortunately unhealthy foods do tend to taste nice and even be addictive and so it is best to try to forget about those. You will enjoy the healthier meals, especially when you start to feel the boost in energy that they give you, but it may just take time for you to adjust to the new way of eating.

It could be a difficult journey. You may find that you crave sugar, you miss your old diet and you really want to go back. You need to work hard to fight against these feelings because you will find that making a change to your diet will have a huge effect on your life. It can affect your health, moods and relationships. It can make you feel much happier, more energetic, less nervous and generally better. Keep this is mind when you are struggling with it.

If you do have a problem, you go back to having those bad foods again, do not punish yourself. You will have already have done that by eating the stuff. Just praise yourself for seeing the error of your ways and feel happy that you have the opportunity to go back to being healthy again. You will have not done yourself massive harm and you can undo any damage that you have done.

Weight and Hypoglycaemia

There is not a standard figure for a hypoglycaemic. With other diseases there is often a classic weight, such as diabetics are normally overweight. However, there are different types with hypoglycaemia.

Underweight

If you often feel sick when you do not eat regularly, then there is a temptation to continue to skip meals. Some hypoglycaemics never have much of an appetite for this reason. High adrenalin can also be a cause of low blood sugar and cause a person to be buzzing all of the time. Always on the move or worrying about things can cause someone to burn off calories and be very thin.

Overweight

Some hypoglycaemics do not get a sick feeling when they miss meals and so they are not averse to eating. In fact if they get food cravings, then they can tend to overeat. Eating a lot of sugary foods can cause blood sugar to spike and dip throughout the day and when it dips, your body may demand food. This means that it can be easy to get overweight.

Cravings

With sensitivity to sugar it can be common to crave sugar. In fact, many people who suffer from hypoglycaemia tend to have a tendency to be addicted to things such as sugar but also alcohol, drugs and things like that. It is therefore important to work hard on balancing the blood sugar to try to stop these unhealthy cravings. They may never be eliminated but as long as you can work hard on getting them down to a minimum, it should help you to fight against them yourself. Of course if you do have a serious problem with a toxic substance then it is sensible to seek medical help as soon as possible.

Trying to ignore cravings can be difficult. If you give in to them, then you could end up eating foods that are not good for you. If you try to ignore them, then you could end up eating great quantities of foods which although they are healthy, can still end up causing you to put on weight. Hopefully, you should find that by sticking to the recommended diet of regular meals and ones that do not spike your blood sugar, then you should not get as many cravings.

Future weight

It is possible that you will find, once you start adding regular snacks in to your diet, that you put on weight. You may have been thin because you did not feel like eating but may find that your appetite has returned. You need to make sure that you do not overeat. Keep main meals a smaller size to allow for the additional calories you are having due to the snacks between meals. Also watch the calories in your drinks, try to avoid high fat milky drinks and things like this.

Exercise can make your blood sugar go too low. However, do not give up exercising, just experiment with different types until you find something that suits you. It is still important to do exercise that raises your heart rate every day and so you could find that you need to eat something just before you exercise it could help. The exercise will help to stop you putting on so much weight as well.

Losing Weight

It can be more difficult to lose weight, because eating less can result in low blood sugar. It is important, therefore to make sure that you are cutting down on the right things. Make sure that you still eat regularly, every three hours. However, reduce things which will not make such a big difference. Reduce the fat a little, have lower fat proteins or just reduce your portion sizes a bit. Gradually cutting down is better, because it will make less of a difference to your blood sugar.

Do not expect big dramatic weight loss. Be patient with yourself and as long as it is creeping down slowly and you are still feeling well, then this is a great result. It is a healthy way to lose weight as well.

If you are having a lot of trouble, then you could get help form your doctor. They should be able to look at what you eat and let you know where to cut down. If you put together a list of what you eat and how much, they will be able to easily identify the changes that you could make.

Case Studies

Changing your diet can have a big difference on your life. Here are a few cases when this has been the case.

Case Study One – Teenage Girl

The girl in question had been identified as having low blood sugar as a baby but was told by the doctor to eat lots of sugar. As a teenager she had trouble sleeping   waking in the night and not being able to go back to sleep. Her mother noticed that it was worse when she had salad for her main meal and went to the doctor and saw a dietician. The dietician recommended a change in diet, cutting out sugar and white flour but the girl tried it a bi and didn't like it. Eventually she started researching it herself and made the changes needed.

The difference was remarkable. Not only was she able to sleep better or when she did wake up, get a snack and then easily get back to sleep, but her whole temperament changed. She was no longer irritable and snappy and also was a lot less nervous and shy.

Case Study Two – Mother of Two

This woman had just given birth to twins. She had low energy levels because she had anaemia and was getting very little sleep and so chose to eat to keep awake. She felt more and more sluggish and could not understand why.

In the end she decided to get her eating back on track by sticking to a diet which has fewer carbohydrates and more proteins and a lot more vegetables, so that she could lose weight. She also exercised a bit more. Not only did she lose weight but her blood sugar balanced and her energy levels went back to normal. She could cope more easily with the sleepless nights.

Case Study Three – Retired Man

This man changed his diet so that he had snacks between meals and worked hard on having no sugar and no white carbohydrates. He became more confident. However, he put on weight because of the extra snacks and so cut them out. He also started lapsing in sticking strictly to the diet and started eating puddings, cakes, biscuits and white rice and pasta at times. He found that his nerves started to play up and he started to get panic attacks.

Curing Hypoglycaemia

There are some books that you can buy which claim that they can cure hypoglycaemia. This sounds fantastic, but it depends exactly what they are referring to. The symptoms can be eliminated, in some cases, if a good lifestyle including sensible diet, regular eating and exercise management; however this is not a cure. Going back to eating sugary foods again is likely to make the symptoms return.

Low Blood Sugar can be caused by a number of reasons, but often the reasons are unknown. This means that finding a cure for the low blood sugar could mean curing the thing that is causing it, whether that is some sort of illness of dysfunction in the body. This is not always possible to do.

It can be great thinking that there could be a cure, where you will be able to adjust your diet for a while and then be able to start eating other things again. It is something that you could try, but it is risky. You may start to get all of those nasty symptoms again and these will not be nice.

You may not notice an occasional change, so if you ate out on an occasion and had white rice with your curry, you may not see a change. However, if you suddenly started eating white carbohydrates and sugar on a regular basis, then you would probably notice the difference.

Research into Hypoglycaemia

The research on hypoglycaemia is very much lacking. There has been a lot of money spent on diabetes and this is because they need medication and so the drug companies pay for the research, to show that their medication works the best. There is medication that can help low blood sugar and so no drug companies fund research. This means that very little research is done. In the UK, it is often not recognised as a disease and so this is another reason why little research is done.

Therefore, the information available about it is very much based on individual sufferers' experiences, rather than factual research. This is why it is important to see whether things work for you or not. Even with medication, some drugs do not work for certain people and so the same thing will apply here.

It can be a good idea to keep a diary, noting down foods, the times you have eaten, exercise done and how you felt. This could help you to identify whether certain foods, eating patterns and exercise has an effect on how you feel.

Every person is an individual and that is what makes us special. It also means that there is no one fit solution for everyone. This explains why two people; both with diabetes may be on different medication. The same applies here and so a diet solution for one person many not work for another due to the severity of their condition, any food allergies and the cause of their hypoglycaemia.

Controlling Blood sugar

So getting rid of the symptoms of hypoglycaemia relies on controlling blood sugar. This means keeping the blood sugar at a stable level throughout the day. This will avoid the spikes and troughs caused by sugary foods and also keep blood sugar generally higher.

Eating regularly is very important. This is why the meal plans have three meals and three snacks. If you leave too long between meals, you will start to see the low blood sugar symptoms appearing. Therefore having breakfast as close to waking a possible, then a snack mid-way between breakfast and lunch, then a snack mid-afternoon and something in the evening before bed. You may need to adjust it slightly depending on when you eat your main meals.

It is best to have food every 2/3 hours. Therefore an example could be :

7am breakfast

9.30am snack

12 lunch

2.30pm snack

5pm dinner

8pm snack

or it may be more like:

8am breakfast

10.30am snack

1pm lunch

3.30pm snack

5pm afternoon tea

8pm supper

It may be more difficult to plan things sometimes. If you are at work, you may only get certain set breaks or things like that. You may also find it embarrassing, always having to eat regularly. If you explain to people, why you are doing it, that it is a medical condition, they should be more understanding rather than thinking you are greedy. Some people do find it hard to eat in public and that might be something that you will have to work on. However you manage it, there is always a way to make sure that you make improvements to your blood sugar, it just takes some careful thought.

It can be wise to carry snacks with you, just in case you feel the symptoms of low blood sugar, especially If you are going to be somewhere that food isn't easily available.

It can be useful to keep a food diary, so that you remember what times you should be eating and even plan out a days food beforehand. This should stop you getting the wrong sorts of food.

It can be difficult to remember at the beginning and you may find yourself accidentally buying or eating foods that you should not be. It can be hard to break a habit, but if you want to feel better, then you will need to.

Awareness of Blood Sugar

Once you start thinking about blood sugar and how you should be eating, it can be difficult not to become obsessed by it. It is good to work hard at eating regularly and having the right foods, but it is also important to stay open minded. A little slip up every now and again will not do too much harm and worrying about it can actually make it a lot worse.

Sometimes we can suddenly become aware that we are late for a meal and notice the low blood sugar symptoms. If we had not been aware of the time we would not have had any symptoms. We are almost panicking suddenly and thinking we should be feeling unwell and so we do so.

So although it is best to stick to regular meals and certain foods, it is a good idea to not completely obsess about it because it can do more harm than good sometimes. If you know you will be in a situation where you will not be able to control what you are eating, you can prepare in several ways. Have a relaxed mind and decide that as there is nothing you can do so just go with the flow. Being stressed with only make the low blood sugar worse. Also carry some snacks with you, leave them in the car or in your bag and you may be able to eat those if you feel unwell. If you think there is a risk that you will have a sever reaction, then have some dextrose tablets with you. Although these will cause a spike in blood sugar, which is what we are trying to avoid, it could help you in this situation where there is no other solution.

In fact it is good to always carry a snack with you. Popping something in the car or your handbag, could b so useful if you feel blood sugar symptoms coming along or you are in a situation where you will be significantly late for a meal or even have to skip one.

Other People and Hypoglycaemia

It can be a little difficult explaining hypoglycaemia to people. Many people will not have heard of it and may not understand that you have a disease when you seem so well. However, there are ways to explain it easily.

It is best to say that you have a sugar intolerance. The word 'intolerance' is easily understood these days and many people say they have food intolerances. You can explain that anything with high amounts of sugar in like cakes and biscuits, sweets, chocolate have to be avoided. Explaining about not eating white carbohydrates van be a little trickier to understand and may be better to only talk about if necessary.

Eating out at other people's houses can be difficult. It is hard to expect them to cater specifically to your needs. One thing that is easy to do is to turn down deserts. If you eat the main meal, which is less likely to affect the blood sugar, then you should be okay. You could also offer to take your own food or supply them with ideas as to what to cook for you.

They may worry, but it is actually quite simple, once you get the hang of it. Sometimes having the odd meal that is not perfectly balanced can be okay, it all depends on you and the severity of your condition.

Conclusion

So, like anything, the 'cure' to your hypoglycaemia will depend on you and how it affects you. You will find that if you can adjust your lifestyle enough, you should be able to feel a lot better, but if you only take a half-hearted approach it may not work as well.

You will need to experiment a bit, in order to find the right approach for you and there is no way that you will be able to go back to eating as you were before and not get the symptoms back. You may want to give it a go, but it is unlikely it will work.

However, the great news is that you can still have an interesting, healthy and varied diet and feel much better. You will be keeping your heart healthy as well as your liver and kidneys and hopefully be protecting yourself against other illnesses while using this approach to eating and you will also feel so much better in yourself.

Good luck with it. Hopefully you will see great and positive changes to your life.

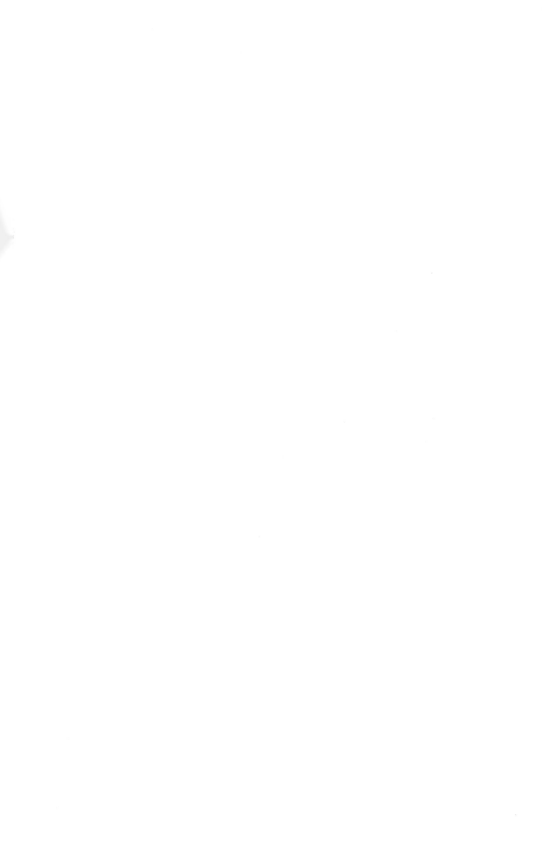

Printed in Great Britain
by Amazon